Out with Gout NOW!

Lee Bradley

DEDICATION

This is for you Sandra for making me smile when my pain was causing me to be a pain.

CONTENTS

Acknowledgments i

1 Gout – Do's and Don'ts 1

2 Gout Myths and Facts 11

3 Gout and PH Levels 13

4 Diary of a Gout Attack

5 Nutrition Guide 16

6 Foods that Lower Uric Acid 25

7 Foods and Inflammation 28

8 Recipes 30

9 My Gout History 45

ACKNOWLEDGMENTS

I would like to express my gratitude to the many people who saw me through this book; to all those who provided support and patience.

1 GOUT OVERVIEW

Basic Review

Gout is a type of arthritis. It occurs when uric acid builds up in blood and causes inflammation in the joints. Acute gout is a painful condition that often affects only one joint; Chronic gout is repeated episodes of pain and inflammation. More than one joint may be affected.

Uric Acid in your blood comes from the breakdown of purine, a substance found in many foods. A high concentration of uric acid in your blood is unhealthy and can lead to various illnesses, both of the ligaments and organs. Diet is the single best way to control how much uric acid makes its way into your body.

Uric Acid and Hyperuricemia

Purines in the liver produce uric acid. The uric acid enters the bloodstream, and most of it eventually goes through the kidneys and is excreted in the urine. The remaining uric acid travels through the intestines, where bacteria help break it down.

Normally these actions keep the level of uric acid in the blood plasma (the liquid part of the blood) at a healthy level, which is below 6.8 mg/dL. But under certain circumstances, the body produces too much uric acid or removes too little. In either case, concentrations of uric acid increase in the blood. This condition is known as *hyperuricemia*.

The levels of uric acid in your blood rise until the level becomes excessive (hyperuricemia), causing urate crystals to build up around the joints. This causes inflammation and severe pain when a gout attack occurs.

Most of the time uric acid dissolves and goes into the urine via the kidneys. However, if the body is producing too much uric acid, or if the kidneys are not excreting enough uric acid, it builds up. The accumulation results in sharp urate crystals which look like needles. They accumulate in the joints or surrounding tissue and cause pain, inflammation and swelling. Fat consumed, tends to bind the uric acid to the kidneys. Stay away from fatty meats, seafood and other fatty products.

Effects

The most common side effect of uric acid build up is gout, which is a painful form of arthritis that millions experience each year. Other complications from excessive uric acid are kidney problems, like kidney stones and even failure of the major organ. Some correlation has been made between high levels of uric acid and high blood pressure as well as heart disease. However, it is unclear if uric acid is a direct contributor to these conditions.

Purine

Purine is a chemical that is found high-fat and oily foods. Organ meats, like liver and kidneys, are high in purine and should be avoid by those who have high uric acid levels. However, it's not just organ meats that are the culprit.

All mammals except humans have an enzyme called *uricase* that breaks down purines so they can be easily removed from the body. In humans, however, purine breaks down into *uric acid*, which is not as easily removed and can build up in body tissues.. Surprisingly, both uric acid and ascorbic acid are strong reducing agents (electron donors) and potent antioxidants. In humans, over half the antioxidant capacity of blood plasma comes from uric acid.

Meats

If you're eating a low purine diet for health reasons, keep in mind that other meats besides those of animal organs can lead to a buildup of uric acid. For a low uric acid diet, any high fat or processed meats, like hot dogs, should be limited. Fatty fishes like mackerel and herring should also be consumed modestly. To fight uric acid, limit your meat consumption to small portions of low fat options, like chicken or lean fish.

Alcohol

Drinking excessive amounts of alcohol can raise your risk of gout. A major 2004 study showed that among alcoholic beverages, beer is the kind of alcohol most strongly linked with gout, followed by spirits. Moderate wine consumption does not appear to increase the risk of developing gout. 5 oz of wine daily can be beneficial. Drinking 2 5 oz glasses daily has no effect and drinking more than 2 glasses can be a gout risk.

Alcohol increases uric acid levels in three ways:
    1. By providing an additional dietary source of purines (the

compounds from which uric acid is formed)
2. By intensifying the body's production of uric acid
3. By interfering with the kidneys' ability to excrete uric acid

Alcohol use is highly associated with gout in younger adults. Binge drinking particularly increases uric acid levels. Alcohol appears to play less of role among elderly patients, especially among women with gout.

Alcohol also raises the lactic acid level in blood, which inhibits uric acid excretion. The higher the daily alcohol intake, the higher the risk of gout . However, differences in risk were observed with different alcoholic drinks. Beer had the greatest effect, probably because of its high purine content, then spirits, whereas wine had no increased risk.

Avoid beer and spirits. Limit wine to more than 2 glasses per day.

Protein
While many meats are not good for your diet if you're watching your uric acid, there are several ways to get your protein without the uric acid. Eggs, low fat milk, and tofu are good selections. These foods will keep your protein levels high, without risking your health.

Fruits and Vegetables
It goes without saying that fruits and vegetables are an important part of any healthy diet. However, if you're working to lower the levels of uric acid in your body, it is essential that you make sure you're getting enough fruits and vegetables. Some vegetables, like peas or beans, are not ideal. Others, like berries, herbs and cherries are good in combating uric acid.

Water
Keeping your body hydrated is important if you want to avoid health complications from uric acid. By drinking at least eight glasses of water each day, you can ensure that toxins are flushed from your system and uric acid buildup is avoided.

Obesity and Age
Researchers report a clear link between body weight and uric acid levels. In one Japanese study, overweight people had two to more than three times the rate of hyperuricemia as those who maintained a healthy weight. Children who are obese may have a higher risk for gout in adulthood.

Gout usually occurs in middle-aged men, peaking in the mid-40s. It is most often associated in this age group with obesity, high blood pressure, unhealthy cholesterol levels, and heavy alcohol use.

If you're obese or over weight, then you need to lose weight. But do it in a healthy way. Avoid quick weight loss diets as this could trigger gout attacks. The nutrition charts and recipes in this book will help you get to a healthy weight and lower your uric acid.

Vitamin C

Vitamin C has a modest uricosuric effect and in the Health Professionals Follow-up Study (HPFS), there was an inverse relationship between vitamin C intake and sUA (serum uric acid). In a randomized placebo-controlled trial, vitamin C supplementation (500 mg/day) for 2 months resulted in a significant reduction in sUA of 0.5 mg/dl (~20% of the starting values)

Uricosuric is the process of increasing the excretion of uric acid in the urine and decreasing the uric acid in the blood.

Fructose

Fructose is known to raise the serum urate level. It is unclear whether this is a particular effect of fructose derived from corn, which is the main sweetener used in the USA, or whether it extends to sucrose (a disaccharide of fructose and glucose), which is the main sweetener used elsewhere in the world. However, the USA does seem to have a particularly strong combination of lifestyle risk factors for primary gout and has led the current pandemic of obesity and metabolic syndrome, perhaps largely explaining the higher increases in incidence and prevalence seen in the USA.

Avoid foods with Fructose while trying to lower uric acid levels. Diet drinks are ok.

Meats and Seafood

Data from the large Health Professionals Follow-up Study (HPFS) have shown that the relative risk of gout is higher in people who eat a high red meat diet: the relative risk of a first attack of gout associated with an additional daily portion of meat was 1.21 (95% CI 1.04, 1.41). Higher consumption of seafood was associated with a lesser, but still significant, increase in risk.

Avoid red meat and seafood.

Purine Rich Vegetables & Low Fat Dairy

Diets high in purine-rich vegetables did not increase the risk, while diets high in low-fat dairy products were associated with reduced risk (relative risk with additional daily serving 0.79; 95% CI 0.71, 0.87) .

Enjoy your low fat dairy as much as you wish. The purine in vegetables is processed differently in your body.

Cherries

There are anecdotal reports that consumption of cherries has a beneficial effect on gout and this is supported by a recent study showing a decrease in urate levels after consumption of cherries but not other fruits. The mechanism for this, and whether it relates to differential vitamin C content, is not clear.

Drink a couple of 8 oz. glasses of cherry juice daily or eat 20-30 cherries daily.

Metabolic syndrome

Hyperuricaemia is an integral part of the metabolic syndrome, together with hypertension, obesity, dyslipidaemia and insulin resistance. One Korean study [1]showed a prevalence of metabolic syndrome (defined by the National Cholesterol Education Program – Adult Treatment Panel criteria) of 44% in gout patients compared with 5% in historical controls. In a US population, the metabolic syndrome (defined by the same criteria) was present in 63% of those with gout compared with 25% of those without gout. In men at increased risk for cardiovascular events, a diagnosis of gout associates with a significantly increased risk of the future development of Type II diabetes, even after adjustment for sUA levels. In the HPFS, obesity, weight gain and hypertension have all been shown to be independent risk factors for the development of gout.

---

[1] Oxford Journals;
http://rheumatology.oxfordjournals.org/content/48/suppl_2/ii2.full

2 GOUT: MYTHS AND FACTS

Myth: Only wealthy and obese people get gout.
Truth: People of all sizes get gout — although extra pounds increase the risk, says John Reveille, M.D., director of rheumatology at the University of Texas Health Science Center in Houston. Gout is also more common in people who have other, often weight-related health problems, including diabetes and high blood pressure or cholesterol. And while income has nothing to do with the condition, genes do play a part: If your parents had gout, you're more likely to have it as well.

Myth: Women aren't afflicted by gout.
Truth: Men and women alike can develop the disease, although men are more vulnerable earlier in life. "Gout is 10 times more common in men than in women, until women reach menopause. The incidence of new cases of gout in men and women tends to equal out after age 60 or so," says Herbert Baraf, M.D., clinical professor of medicine at George Washington University Medical Center in Washington, D.C.

Myth: Gout pain always attacks the big toe.
Truth: Gout occurs when uric acid builds up in the blood, forming crystals that lodge in and inflame joints. It's true that gout often first attacks the joints of the big toe, but it can also occur in the knees, ankles, feet and hands. In women with osteoarthritis, for example, gout pain commonly starts in the small joints of the hands. Although the first attacks often involve only one or two joints, over time multiple joints become affected. If the disease isn't treated, it can cause permanent damage.

Myth: If you stay away from liver and alcohol, you'll avoid gout attacks.
Truth: Alcoholic drinks — especially beer — and organ meats such as liver and some fish, including anchovies and sardines, are very high in purines. When the body breaks down purines it creates uric acid, so eating a lot of purine-rich foods does increase the risk of an attack. But while avoiding these foods may reduce attacks, it won't halt them, says Reveille.

Myth: Gout is painful, but it won't kill you.
Truth: Gout can't kill you directly, but it can cause serious health problems that may eventually kill you, says Robert Keenan, M.D., assistant professor of medicine at Duke University. It can increase your risk of a heart attack or stroke, and it also may be linked to insulin resistance, the body's shrinking ability to use insulin to lower blood sugar. If gout is untreated, you can

develop clumps of uric acid crystals called tophi, which can become infected and life threatening.

Myth: There aren't effective medicines for gout.
Truth: Many medications put the brakes on gout. Some control pain and inflammation immediately and others get at the root cause by eliminating the deposited uric acid crystals. Colchicine (Colcrys) is prescribed for acute gout flare-ups. A plant extract, it's been used to treat gout for 2,000 years. Colchicine works within several minutes to several hours to block gout inflammation. The sooner you start it, the more likely the attack will resolve quickly. An injected steroid also tackles inflammation, usually controlling pain and swelling within 24 hours. Prescription drugs such as allopurinol (Lopurin, Zyloprim), febuxostat (Uloric) and probenecid (Benemid) all alleviate gout by controlling blood levels of uric acid. Also, two years ago the FDA approved an intravenous drug for people with advanced gout — pegloticase (Krystexxa) — that lowers uric acid levels and reduces deposits of uric acid crystals in the joints and soft tissue. Most people who have gout will need to be on a uric-acid-lowering drug for life, usually just one or two pills a day.

Myth: Once you've got gout, lifestyle changes don't really help.
Truth: Lifestyle changes can reduce both the severity and frequency of attacks. For starters, when people lose weight, they often have fewer attacks, says Reveille.

Animal proteins have a higher level of purines, so it's better to eat vegetable proteins like beans and peas.

In fact, a 2010 review in the rheumatology journal Current Opinion in Rheumatology notes that protein-rich foods such as dairy products, nuts, beans, peas and whole grains are healthy choices for people with gout, reducing the risk of heart disease and possibly lowering the risk of insulin resistance.

You need to abstain from alcohol during the first six months of treatment, until medications have stabilized uric acid levels. After that, it's fine to drink — in moderation.

3 GOUT AND YOUR BODY'S PH LEVEL

How Does pH Affect Gout?

If you cannot get rid of uric acid formed in the blood during the breakdown of certain foods, the crystalline waste product may cause kidney stones or painful gout in joints. Since high amounts of uric acid levels register correspondingly low pH, the pH of blood and urine would seem to have a direct relationship to gout formation. Only your doctor can tell if your symptoms indicate gout and what treatment is best once gout is diagnosed.

Uric Acid Level

The high concentration of uric acid in your blood, also known as hyperuricemia, comes from your body processing the purine found in a variety of foods. MayoClinic.com states that excessive uric acid, which registers at below pH levels of 7, may be excreted through the urine without adverse effect, but some people cannot process the low pH uric acid and suffer bouts of gout, chronic kidney disease or even heart disease.

Causes of Uric Acid Production

High levels of uric acid in the blood are in inverse relation to pH levels, with the higher uric acid levels registering lower pH values. MayoClinic.com states that the causes of not being able to process uric acid may be from either overproduction of uric acid in the blood or poor elimination of the uric acid in urine. Causal factors include family history of gout, diuretic medication, high caffeine intake and a diet that includes organ meat, herring or legumes.

Neutralize pH

You can cut down on the amount of low pH uric acid formed in the blood by attempting to neutralize pH values through diet and exercise. The University of Maryland Medical Center advises you drink 6 to 8 glasses of water daily to avoid the dehydration that may trigger a gout attack. The site also advises avoiding alcohol and tobacco use and performing at least a half-hour of brisk walking, swimming or cycling daily to help flush uric acid through your body.

Unknown Factors

While healthy dieting and exercise are always good courses of action, there is much still unknown about the relationship of low pH, high uric acid and gout crystals forming in joints. MayoClinic.com states that it is still uncertain whether the low pH, high uric acid found in blood is a direct cause of gout or only an early warning sign of the possibility that gout may be in your future.

How Does Your pH Level Actually Work?

If you don't know anything about pH readings then this is how it goes... pH runs on a scale from 0-14 with 7 being the neutral level (right in the middle). Any reading below 7 is acidic and anything above 7 is alkaline. Our bodies absolutely <u>must</u> be kept alkaline at all times (7.35-7.45 to be exact) for perfect health. And what's significant in regards to natural remedies for gout is <u>this condition simply cannot occur in an alkaline environment.</u>

It's virtually impossible!

But gout will definitely occur and flourish very nicely in an acidic environment. In fact the main culprit of gout, a build up of uric acid, actually loves it when the body is acidic (probably because it is also an acid). But even worse than this is killer diseases such as cancer also grow and thrive in an acidic environment.

So to test your pH level all you have to do is purchase some test strips from your local health food store and follow the instructions. These strips are very simple to use and really are worth their weight in gold!

Some Easy Way's to Increase Your pH Level...

Natural Remedies for Gout pH Booster #1 - Apple Cider Vinegar and Baking Powder:

If you are suffering from a bout of gout right now then one of the quickest ways to alkalize your body is with a combination of organic apple cider vinegar (must contain the mother apple) and baking powder. Take two to three tablespoons of apple cider vinegar (ACV) with ½ a teaspoon of aluminium free baking powder twice a day, 20-30 minutes before each meal. This is a sure fire way to get rid of your gout symptoms, usually within a day or two. (If you find having them on an empty stomach gives you diarrhoea then simply take with your meal instead).

4 THE DIARY OF A GOUT ATTACK

Monday, 8am: I arrive at work feeling really good. I have had very little joint pain over the last few days. It might be safe to eat a hamburger at lunch. I have taken my medicine today, so why not?

12:45pm: I decide to go to McDonald's for lunch. I haven't been there for a while, and it is just across the parking lot from my store. I order 2 double cheeseburgers and a fry. I carry the food back to the store and get a coke out of the machine. On the way back to work, I have a cup of coffee.

4:17pm: I feel a twinge in my left big toe, and my ankle is a little stiff. I just ignore it as another little flare up of Osteo-arthritis. I take a couple of ibuprofen with a sip of water and keep working.

5:12pm: Driving home now. I can't seem to get my left leg and foot comfortable. It feels sore and stiff.

5:35pm: I arrive home, and I struggle with the onset of stiffness and slight pain as I try to move my leg out of the truck. Although it doesn't hurt badly, it is sore enough to keep me from standing up straight. "Now what?" I think to myself. I limp to the house, taking care not to let my dog knock me off balance.

I do some quick chores around the house before I settle in. Walking around seems to loosen my joints up a little and it begins to feel better.

6:19pm: I finally sit down and take off my shoes. It is hard to bend my knee to take off my sock. My toes on my left foot are puffy and my big toe is a little red. I hobble into the kitchen and take three ibuprofen with a glass of wine. I go in and sit down on the living room couch and visit with my wife. After a while, I drift off to sleep.

6:59pm: My wife calls me for dinner. I put my feet on the floor to stand up and I feel more pain in my ankle and toe. Trudging through it, I limp to the dinner table, where I find a sumptuous fare consisting of chicken leg quarters, broccoli and mashed potatoes. There is a leafy green salad with spring greens and fresh spinach.

After dinner, I sit down in the living room to watch a movie with my wife and then the news.

11:30pm: She goes off to bed and I go to my office to check my email, blogs, and my E-bay activities. As I try to get up, I realize that the inactivity has caused my stiffness and pain to worsen. I go to the medicine chest and grab my bottle of Colchicine I take when an attack flares up. The bottle is empty. I take an extra Allopurinol instead, along with 4 Aleve.

I settle in at my desk and do what I need to do. I pour myself a glass of wine.

Tuesday, 12:20am: I turn around in my desk chair and attempt to stand up. The pain and stiffness is worsening. It is becoming more and more difficult to stand and walk, but I still manage to make it to bed. I fall asleep quickly.

2:42am: I am suddenly awakened by the intense pain in my left big toe. It was as if someone snuck into the room and hit me on the toe with a hammer. The pain is excruciating. I try to stand up, but I can't. I do it anyway and try to walk it off. The pain is incredibly intense, but soon it subsides down to an annoying ache. The big toe is red and swollen; the skin is shiny and warm. My ankle and knee are becoming stiffer now. My wife asks me if I took my Colchicine, and I tell her that the bottle was empty, I forgot to refill it. She calls me an idiot, and gets me a Vicodin and a glass of water. I try to go back to sleep. Thank God I go in late in the morning.

8:30am: I wake up and try to stand up. The pain and swelling are incredible now. My head is a little fuzzy from the Vicodin, but a cup of coffee helps to knock that out. I force myself to walk because I can't miss anymore days because of gout.

9:00am: I shower off and struggle getting dressed. It is hard balancing on one foot to put underwear and pants on, let alone trying to bend my knee to put on shoes and socks. My wife packs my lunch, leftovers from last night, and I am off to work.

10:22am: I arrive at work. My whole leg from the knee down is pounding from pain and stiffness. I park my truck close to the door and take my time going in. I grab a shopping cart and use it for a walker; in the hopes that I can loosen my leg up before I reach the time clock.

10:29am: I am at the time clock and I am leaning against a pallet waiting for the time to click over. Once I clock in, I hobble as fast as I can to my department and prepare for work. My boss sees me and notices I am in pain.

"Gout, again?" he asks.

"Yes." I say.

"You'll never get promoted with your health the way it is." And he walks off.

10:33am: I pop the first of two Vicodin that I brought with me today. It will numb my pain enough until I get loosened up.

The next four and a half hours drag on. The pain is incredible, but dulled by the Vicodin. I refrain from using the saw as much as I can while on these meds, lest I lose a finger.

3:00pm: Lunchtime. I take my lunch to the break room and finish it off quickly. Afterwards, I hobble out to my truck and take a 40 minute nap before returning to work, but I am unable to sleep because of the pain and other discomfort. Again, the inactivity has made everything stiffer and more painful.

3:55pm: I hobble back into the store and take the second Vicodin and an Allopurinol. I have a cup of coffee and try to keep working as best as I can.

7:30pm: I am finally off work, and near tears with pain. I nearly crawl to the truck and climb in for a painful drive home.

8:07pm: I arrive home, and again struggle to get out of the truck. As I do, Wyatt, my 80lb Labrador is so happy to see me, he jumps up and lands on my big toe with all of his weight. I hit the ground writhing in extreme pain as Wyatt (the big oaf) licks my face. Once I am composed, I crawl on all fours to the truck and pull myself up, and I hobble slowly to the side door of the living room. I climb up the steps, walk in and collapse on the couch. Pepper, the Aussie that lives indoors begins licking my face.

8:12pm: My wife comes in and helps me to take off my shoes. She is taken aback by the size of my red, shiny and swollen foot and toes.

"Del, this is a bad one." She says. "Did you pick up the Colchicine today?"

"I thought you were going to do it." I said.

"You are such an idiot!" She went on. "You have a pharmacy where you work!"

"Yeah but it's cheaper if you get it at Kroger." I said.

She brought my dinner to me on the couch, called me an idiot a couple of more times, and then sat down. I didn't move from the couch until I went to bed.

10:45pm: I took another Vicodin and crawled (literally) to bed (Pepper thought it was playtime). The Vicodin put me to sleep quickly.

Wednesday, 6:00am: The alarm sounds, and I try to get up. There is no freaking way can I stand up, no matter how hard I push myself. The pain was 15 on a scale of 1 to 10. I reached for the phone and called out for the day. My boss was not happy. I had no more sick time left.

9:35am: My wife returned from the pharmacy with my Colchicine. I took two of them right away and then one each hour until I was relieved, or diarrhea sets in. I stay off my feet all day.

4:00pm: By now I am able to walk comfortably to the bathroom to get the kaopectate. My wife is beginning to cook dinner, and I see that she is preparing salmon with asparagus and a dark leafy green salad.

She offers me a glass of wine, and I turn it down. I also turned down dinner, as I did not want a replay of the events of the last two days.

Thursday, 10:13am: I wake up, nearly pain free. I am off today, and I am going to take it easy, and this time I swear that from now on, I will eat and drink more responsibly!

6:15pm: A friend comes over with a 12 pack of beer. I think "Why not? I have a fresh bottle of Colchicine!"

Epilogue: I missed three more days of work. Having gout is a life changing experience, and if you aren't willing to go with the changes and be aware of what you put into your body, you will forever suffer the painful consequences.

Below is a sample of a daily diary. This can be downloaded from the OutWithGout website.

---

[2] Del Banks - http://badegg.hubpages.com/hub/The-Diary-of-a-Gout-Attack

Gout Daily Diary

Date:

Time	Food and Drink	Activities – Work, Weather, Sleep	Medication – Dose	Pain and Other Symptoms

5 PURINE INFLAMMATORY CHART

About the Chart

I created this chart to assist you in determining foods purine content and the inflammation content. I feel combining the both is very important in fighting off gout.

For purines, the higher the purine content, the more it contributes to gout. For the inflammation factor, the higher the number, the better the food is for you at fighting inflammation. Try and keep your net Inflammation Rating to a net 50 or more for the day.

It's not always possible to choose a food with both low purine and a high IF number. Always go with the low purine content since that directly affects the uric acid levels.

Purine Inflammation Chart

Name	Purine	Uric Acid	IF Rating	Glycemic
Yeast	285	684	27	1
Cannery Row	200	480	135	0
Trout	144	345	153	0
Sardine	140	336	763	0
Calf liver	120	288	-130	3
Goose	106	254	63	0
Pork	88	210	-15	0
Ham	85	204	30	2
Soybean meat	123	296	-44	6
Soy Powder	110	265	-10	1
Tofu	29	70	0	2
Soy sauce	25	60	4	1
Chickpeas	46	109	-127	23
White beans	18	42	-105	25
Peas green	40	95	5	33
Raisins dried	45	107	-557	75
Wheat flour	16	38	-101	15

Beans green	18	42	10	2
Peanut	33	79	127	0
Hazelnut	15	37	437	0
Pumpkin-seeds	36	85	-142	2
Almond	15	37	278	0
Poppy	71	170	-19	0
Sesame seeds	26	62	41	0
Sunflower seeds	60	143	17	0
Walnut	10	25	-158	0
Pineapple	8	20	65	6
Apple Raw	6	15	-20	3
Apple dried	25	60	-193	26
Orange	8	20	9	6
Apricot	8	20	3	6
Apricot dried	31	73	-227	40
Eggplant	8	20	-4	1
Avocado	13	30	181	4
Banana	24	57	-115	7
Pear	5	12	-30	5
Blackberry	6	15	6	4
Date	21	50	-416	57
Strawberry	9	21	28	3
Figs dried	27	64	-322	44
Grapefruit	6	15	18	7
Raspberry	8	18	1	3
Melon	14	33	76	5
Cherry	7	17	-47	7
Kiwi	8	19	34	8
Cucumber	3	6	0	1
Pumpkin	3	7	65	3
Peppers green	4	10	47	2
Peppers red	6	15	126	3
Peach	9	21	-25	5
Plum	10	24	-366	54
Plum dried	27	64	-366	54

Cranberry	5	13	-21	5
Tomato	4	9	14	2
Watermelon	8	20	-7	3
Grape	11	27	-33	5
Zucchini	8	20	7	2
Jalapenos	Low	Low	342	2
Red Chili Peppers	Low	Low	274	2

6 FOODS THAT LOWER URIC ACID

Water
Water flushes out toxins including excess uric acid from the body. Have at least 10- 12 glasses of water daily.

Cherries
Cherries have anti - inflammatory substances named anthocyanis that help reduce uric acid levels .It prevents the uric acid from crystallizing and being deposited in the joints. Cherries also neutralize the acids and help prevent inflammation and pain. 200 gms per day is very effective in bringing down uric acid.

You can also substitute 2 8oz glasses of cherry juice a day. This is what I prefer.

Berries

Berries especially strawberries, and blueberries have anti-inflammatory properties so include them in your diet.

Apple
Malic acid in apple neutralizes uric acid and thus provides relief to the sufferers. You should consume one apple daily after a meal.

Lime
The citric acid found in lime is a solvent of the uric acid .The juice of half a lime squeezed into a glass of water should be taken twice daily.

French bean juice
Another effective home remedy for gout is French beans juice. The healthy juice can be consumed twice everyday for treating gout or high uric acid.

Celery seed
This is a popular home remedy to lower uric acid levels in the body. Have celery seeds extract to get best results.

Apple cider vinegar
Drink apple cider vinegar. Add 3 teaspoons of vinegar to 8 ounces of water and have it 2-3 times every day to treat uric acid.

Pinto beans
A diet rich in folic acid can help lower uric acid naturally. Folic acid rich foods like pinto beans, sunflower seeds and lentils should be included in your diet.

Vegetable juices
Carrot juice in combination with beet and cucumber juice is also very effective .100 ml each of beet juice and cucumber juice should be mixed with 300 ml carrot juice and taken daily.

Low fat dairy products like milk, curd help lower uric acid level.

Foods rich in Vit C
Include vitamin C rich foods & supplements in your daily diet to reduce uric acid in the body. It disintegrates uric acid and forces it out of the body through urine. Good sources of vitamin C are awla, guava, kiwi, sweet lime, oranges, capsicum, lemon, tomato and green leafy vegetables.

High-fiber foods
According to the University of Maryland Medical Center, adding foods high in dietary fiber may help lower uric acid levels in your blood. Dietary fiber may help absorb uric acid in your bloodstream, allowing it to be eliminated from your body through your kidneys. Increase the consumption of dietary soluble fibers such as Isabgol, Oats, Broccoli , apples, oranges, pears, strawberries, blueberries, cucumbers, celery, and carrots , barley .

Bananas are also beneficial in lowering uric acid

Green tea
Consume green tea on a regular basis to control hyperuricemia (high uric acid levels) and lower your risk of developing gout.

Grains and Vegetables
Eating grains that are more alkaline such as jowar,bajra are helpful.

Tomatoes, broccoli, and cucumbers are some of the veggies that you need to start including in your meals. Tomatoes are one of the best vegetables that you could have for lowering uric acid. Fresh tomato is alkaline by nature and when it is exposed to the blood stream it increases the alkalinity of the blood

Raw vegetables like potatoes or corns are effective to reduce uric acid in the body. Have them raw or steam these vegetables.

7 – FOODS AND INFLAMMATION

Inflammation: [3]A localized physical condition in which part of the body becomes reddened, swollen, hot and often painful, especially as a reaction to injury or infection.

We all know when something is inflamed. But, what about inflammation on the inside of our bodies? Internal inflammation can happen for a host of different reasons: high temperatures when cooking food, eating processed foods, sugar, trans fats, etc. A high level of inflammation within the body can cause many health problems. An easy way to combat this? Eat more anti-inflammatory foods and eliminate the inflammatory ones.

But, what is an anti-inflammatory food? More importantly, what is an inflammatory food? While you know healthy, whole foods from processed foods, none of us can see the true effect they have on our bodies (sometimes, until it's too late).

Often diseases such as diabetes, PCOS, excess weight gain, coronary heart disease and countless other illnesses can be contributed to the inflammation from various foods.

TOP 10 ANTI-INFLAMMATORY FOODS

1. **Wild Alaskan Salmon**: Salmon contains anti-inflammatory omega-3s (wild is better than farmed) and has been known to help numerous ailments. Try and incorporate oily fish into your diet twice weekly. If you don't like fish, try a high quality fish supplement.

2. **Kelp**: High in fiber, this brown algae extract helps control liver and lung cancer, douses inflammation, and is anti-tumor and anti-oxidative. Kombu, wakame and arame are good sources.

3. **Extra Virgin Olive Oil**: The secret to longevity in Mediterranean culture, this oil provides a healthy dose of fats that fights inflammation, can help lower risks of asthma and arthritis, as well as protect the heart and blood vessels.

---

[3] Rea Frey; http://www.chicagonow.com/clean-convenient-cuisine/2010/09/best-and-worst-top-10-most-inflammatory-and-anti-inflammatory-foods/

4. **Cruciferous Vegetables**: Broccoli, brussel sprouts, kale and cauliflower are all loaded with antioxidants. Naturally detoxifying, they can help rid the body of possible harmful compounds.

5. **Blueberries**: Blueberries not only reduce inflammation, but they can protect the brain from aging and prevent diseases, such as cancer and dementia. Aim for organic berries, as pesticides are hard to wash away due to their size.

6. **Turmeric**: This powerful Asian spice contains a natural anti-inflammatory compound, curcumin, which is often found in curry blends. It is said to have the same effect as over-the counter pain relievers (but without their side effects).

7. **Ginger**: Ginger contains a host of health benefits. Among them, it helps reduce inflammation and control blood sugar. Ginger tea is a great addition to any diet.
8. **Garlic**: Though a little more inconsistent (in terms of research), garlic can help reduce inflammation, regulate glucose and help your body fight infection.

9. **Green Tea**: Like produce, this tea contains anti-inflammatory flavonoids that may even help reduce the risks of certain cancers.

10. **Sweet Potato**: A great source of complex carbs, fiber, beta-carotene, manganese and vitamin B6 and C, these potatoes actually help heal inflammation in the body.

TOP 10 INFLAMMATORY FOODS

These foods have been linked to obesity, increased risks of numerous diseases and even death in some cases.

1. **Sugar:** Sugar is everywhere. Try and limit processed foods, desserts and snacks with excess sugar. Opt for fruit instead.

2. **Common Cooking Oils**: Safflower, soy, sunflower, corn, and cottonseed. These oils promote inflammation and are made with cheaper ingredients.

3. **Trans Fats**: Trans fats increase bad cholesterol, promote inflammation, obesity and resistance to insulin. They are in fried foods, fast foods,

commercially baked goods, such as peanut butter and items prepared with partially hydrogenated oil, margarine and vegetable oil.

4. **Dairy**: While kefir and some yogurts are acceptable, dairy is hard on the body. Milk is a common allergen that can trigger inflammation, stomach problems, skin rashes, hives and even breathing difficulties.

5. **Feedlot-Raised Meat**: Animals who are fed with grains like soy and corn contain high inflammation. These animals also gain excess fat and are injected with hormones and antibiotics. Always opt for organic, free-range meats who have been fed natural diets.

6. **Red and Processed Meat**: Red meat contains a molecule that humans don't naturally produce called Neu5GC. Once you ingest this compound, your body develops antibodies which may trigger constant inflammatory responses. Reduce red meat consumption and replace with poultry, fish and learn cuts of red meat, once a week at most.

7. **Alcohol**: Regular consumption of alcohol causes irritation and inflammation to numerous organs, which can lead to cancer.

8. **Refined Grains**: "Refined" products have no fiber and have a high glycemic index. They are everywhere: white rice, white flour, white bread, pasta, pastries... Try and replace with minimally processed grains.

9. **Artificial Food Additives**: Aspartame and MSG are two common food additives that can trigger inflammation responses. Try and omit completely from the diet.

10. **Fill in the Blank**: Do you constantly have headaches or feel tired? Sometimes, you may develop an allergy to a food and not even know it. Coffee, certain vegetables, cheese... there might be a trigger you aren't even aware of. Try and take a few foods out to see how you feel and slowly incorporate them back in to see if there might be a hidden culprit lurking in your diet!

8 RECIPES

About the Recipes
The recipes included are based on a low purine diet. All recipes are low impact to gout. Staying on a low purine diet is very difficult. It means limiting what you can eat. So hopefully these recipes will be as tasty for you as they are for me.

Walnut-Grain Burgers

These burgers are packed will belly-flattening monounsaturated fats. For superfast meals, keep cooked, cooled burgers frozen for up to 3 months. Simply microwave to reheat.

What you'll need:
2 cups instant brown rice
1 3/4 cups low-sodium vegetable broth
1/2 onion, finely chopped
1 carrot, finely chopped
2 cloves garlic
1 1/4 cups walnuts
1 egg white
1 tablespoon salt-free seasoning blend
1/2 cup sesame seeds paprika
10 reduced-calorie hamburger buns
10 slices tomato
10 lettuce leaves

How to make it:
1. Combine the rice, broth, onion, carrot, and garlic in a large saucepan. Cover and bring to a boil over high heat. Reduce the heat so the mixture simmers. Cook for 5 minutes. Remove from the heat and set aside, covered, for 5 minutes. Spread on a baking sheet to cool.

2. Process the walnuts in the bowl of a food processor fitted with a metal blade until finely ground. Add the rice mixture, egg white, and seasoning. Pulse until the mixture sticks together. With wet hands, roll into 10 balls and then flatten into patties. Place the sesame seeds on a shallow plate and press the patties into them. Sprinkle with the paprika.

3. Coat a nonstick griddle or large skillet with cooking spray and heat over medium heat. Cook the patties for about 3 minutes or until golden. Turn carefully and cook for about 4 minutes longer or until heated through. Place each patty on a bun with a tomato slice and lettuce leaf.

Makes 10 servings. *Per serving: 30 1.5 cal, 14.7 g fat (1.6 g sat), 38.2 g carbs, 6 g fiber, 217.7 mg sodium, 10.4 g protein*

Curried Carrot, Sweet Potato, and Ginger Soup

This soup gets its wonderfully creamy texture from puréed carrots and sweet potatoes rather than cream, a dairy product Willett discourages due to its high saturated-fat content.

Ingredients

- 2 teaspoons canola oil
- 1/2 cup chopped shallots
- 3 cups (1/2-inch) cubed peeled sweet potato
- 1 1/2 cups (1/4-inch) sliced peeled carrots
- 1 tablespoon grated ginger
- 2 teaspoons curry powder
- 3 cups fat-free, less-sodium chicken broth
- 1/2 teaspoon salt

Preparation

Heat oil in a large saucepan over medium-high heat. Add shallots; saute 3 minutes or until tender. Add potato, carrots, ginger, and curry; cook 2 minutes. Add broth; bring to a boil. Cover, reduce heat, and simmer 25 minutes or until vegetables are tender; stir in salt.

Pour half of soup in a food processor; pulse until smooth. Repeat procedure with remaining soup.

Makes 5 servings. *Per serving: 144 cal, 2.5g fat (0.2g sat), 27.3g carbs, 3.9g fiber, 531 mg sodium, 4.1 g protein, chol 0.0mg*

Waldorf Salad

Fill up on this healthy, fresh salad filled with crisp fruit and vegetables. Spare the fat with fat-free mayonnaise and indulge even more.

Prep Time: 10 minutes; Yield: Makes 4 servings (serving size: 1/2 cup salad and 2 boston or bibb lettuce leaves)

Ingredients

- 2 tablespoons low-fat mayonnaise
- 1 tablespoon lemon juice
- 2 small (Gala or Fuji) apples, cubed
- 1 cup seedless red grapes, halved
- 1/3 cup dried cranberries
- 1/4 cup coarsely chopped walnuts
- 1/4 cup thinly sliced celery (about 1 stalk)
- 8 Boston or Bibb lettuce leaves
-

Preparation

1. Combine mayonnaise and lemon juice in a medium bowl. Add apples, grapes, and cranberries; mix well.

2. Add the walnuts and celery, and mix well. Serve it on a bed of 2 lettuce leaves. The salad can be refrigerated up to 2 hours before serving.

Nutrition: *Per serving: 153 cal, 6g fat (1g sat), 26g carbs, 3g fiber, 72mg sodium, 2g protein, chol 0.0mg*

Tomato Crostini

Choose this tasty recipe to serve hungry guests as they arrive; it won't ruin their appetite or leave them in major gout pain. What's more, this simple appetizer uses plum tomatoes, which are better than most other varieties in the winter.

Yield: 2 servings (serving size: 2 bread slices and about 1/3 cup tomato mixture)

Ingredients

- 1/2 cup chopped plum tomato
- 1 tablespoon chopped fresh basil
- 1 tablespoon chopped pitted green olives
- 1 teaspoon capers
- 1/2 teaspoon balsamic vinegar
- 1/2 teaspoon olive oil
- 1/8 teaspoon sea salt
- Dash of freshly ground black pepper
- 1 garlic clove, minced
- 4 (1-inch-thick) slices French bread baguette
- Cooking spray
- 1 garlic clove, halved
-

Preparation

1. Preheat oven to 375°.
2. Combine first 9 ingredients.
3. Lightly coat both sides of bread slices with cooking spray; arrange bread slices in a single layer on a baking sheet. Bake at 375° for 4 minutes on each side or until lightly toasted.
4. Rub 1 side of bread slices with halved garlic; top evenly with tomato mixture.

Nutrition: *Per serving: 109cal, 2.8g fat (1.5g sat), 18g carbs, 1.4g fiber, 373mg sodium, 3.1g protein, chol 0.0mg*

Warm Eggplant and Goat Cheese Sandwiches

Eggplant and tomatoes are low-purine foods that blend deliciously with creamy goat cheese for a savory sandwich that packs anything but boring for lunch.

Eggplant is rich in disease-fighting antioxidants. Try a multigrain roll for a fiber boost. To boot, veggies tend to be alkaline (the opposite of acidic), meaning they may help neutralize uric acid.

Ingredients

- 1 teaspoon olive oil
- 2 (1/4-inch) vertical slices small eggplant
- Cooking spray
- 1/4 teaspoon salt
- 1/4 teaspoon freshly ground black pepper
- 1/4 cup (2 ounces) goat cheese, softened
- 2 (1 1/2-ounce) rustic sandwich rolls
- 2 (1/4-inch) slices tomato
- 1 cup arugula

Preparation

1. Preheat oven to 275°.
2. Brush oil over eggplant.
3. Heat a large nonstick skillet coated with cooking spray over medium-high heat. Add eggplant; cook 5 minutes on each side or until lightly browned. Sprinkle with salt and pepper.
4. Spread about 1 tablespoon of goat cheese over cut side of each roll half. Place rolls on a baking sheet, cheese sides up; bake at 275° for 8 to 10 minutes or until thoroughly heated.
5. Remove from oven; top bottom half of each roll with 1 eggplant slice, 1 tomato slice, and 1/2 cup arugula. Top sandwiches with top halves of rolls.

Nutrition: *Per serving: 299 cal, 11.1g fat (5.1g sat), 40g carbs, 9g fiber, 647mg sodium, 12g protein, chol 13mg*

Lemon-and-Sage Roasted Chicken

Although meat is generally a no-no food for people with gout, you can't always avoid it, especially when you're cooking for a group. But you can choose chicken or duck, which have less purine than red meat, pork, and turkey.

This easy recipe enhances the flavors of roasted chicken with lemon and sage. The roasted parsnips, carrots, and turnips on the side are rich in flavor, not purine!

Prep Time: 30 minutes: Yield: Makes 4 servings (plus leftovers) (serving size: 1/8 of chicken and 1/2 cup roasted vegetables)

Ingredients

- 2 lemons, thinly sliced
- 6 fresh sage leaves
- 1 (6-pound) chicken
- 3 teaspoons olive oil, divided
- 3/4 pound parsnips, peeled and trimmed
- 3/4 pound carrots, peeled and trimmed
- 1/2 pound turnips, peeled and trimmed
- 1 pound fingerling potatoes, halved
- 2 tablespoons chopped fresh thyme

Preparation

Preheat oven to 425°. Place 6 lemon slices and sage leaves under skin of chicken. Put remaining lemon into cavity. Tie legs together with twine, and tuck wings under. Brush 1 teaspoon oil over chicken. Place chicken in roasting pan; roast in lower third of oven for 1 hour 15 minutes or until an instant-read thermometer registers 165°. Transfer chicken to a cutting board; let rest for 15 minutes. Meanwhile, cut root vegetables into matchsticks. Toss with potatoes in a baking pan with remaining oil and thyme. Roast, stirring occasionally, for 45 minutes or until tender. 3. Remove skin from chicken. Discard lemons from cavity. Slice enough chicken to serve 4 (such as breasts), and serve with half of vegetables.

Nutrition: *Per serving: 292 cal, 5g fat (1g sat), 22g carbs, 4g fiber, 120mg sodium, 37g protein, chol 96mg*

Zesty Zucchini Spaghetti

Pasta makes a great, low-purine way to get full without the meat. The shredded zucchini and chipotle chiles (roasted jalepeños) give this dish a helping of zest without the purine.

Just be sure to stick to the serving size so you don't get too many calories— being overweight is a risk factor for gout.

Choose whole wheat pasta for a boost of fiber and heart-healthy complex carbohydrates. Fiber keeps you feeling full longer than white pasta.

Yield: Serves 4 (serving size: about 2 cups)

Ingredients

- 3/4 pound uncooked spaghetti
- 1 (7-ounce) can chipotle chiles in adobo sauce
- 2 teaspoons olive oil
- 2 garlic cloves, minced
- 4 cups shredded zucchini (about 1 1/4 pounds)
- 3/4 teaspoon salt
- 1/4 teaspoon black pepper
- 2 tablespoons Parmesan cheese, shaved

Preparation

Cook pasta according to package directions, omitting salt and fat. Remove 1 chile (smaller for less spice, larger for more) and 1 tablespoon sauce from can (reserve remaining sauce for another use). Remove seeds from chile (for extra heat, leave seeds in); mince chile. Heat oil in a large nonstick skillet over medium-high heat. Add chile, sauce, and garlic; sauté 1 minute. Add zucchini; cook, stirring constantly, 4 minutes. Toss pasta with zucchini mixture. Sprinkle with salt, pepper, and cheese.

Nutrition: *Per serving: 386 cal, 5g fat (1g sat), 72g carbs, 5g fiber, 267mg sodium, 14g protein, chol 2mg*

Rosemary-Roasted New Potatoes

Potatoes make for another yummy, satisfying, and low-purine food that is also rich in uric-acid-reducing vitamin C. The fresh rosemary adds a punch of flavor, and is thought to improve circulation—a benefit that could ease gout-related pain and inflammation.

Serve these piping hot seasoned potatoes as a side dish to any kind of chicken, beef or fish meal. They're hearty and seasoned to perfection.

Yield: Makes 4 servings (serving size: about 3/4 cup)

Ingredients

- 1 (1-pound, 4-ounce) package refrigerated red potato wedges (such as Simply Potatoes)
- 2 tablespoons chopped fresh rosemary
- 3 garlic cloves, crushed
- 1 tablespoon olive oil
- 1/2 teaspoon onion powder
- 1/4 teaspoon salt
- 1/4 teaspoon pepper
-

Preparation

Preheat oven to 500°. In a large bowl, combine potatoes and remaining ingredients. Toss thoroughly to coat each potato wedge with oil and seasonings. Place the potato wedges on a baking sheet that's lined with foil. Bake 22 minutes or until tender and golden. Serve hot.

Nutrition: *Per serving: 123 cal, 3g fat (0.5g sat), 19g carbs, 4g fiber, 220mg sodium, 4g protein, chol 0.0mg*

Peaches With Berry Sauce

Instead of the usual chocolate syrup, pour this berry sauce over low-fat vanilla ice cream for a twist on a classic dessert. Dark berries, like the blackberries in this sauce, have been found to lower uric-acid levels in the body.

Plus fruits like peaches and berries are a delicious, low-purine way to satisfy your sweet tooth.

Liven up your vanilla ice cream with an antioxidant-rich berry sauce. Instead of hot fudge or whipped cream, this berry sauce is healthy and sweet without all the calories.

Yield: Makes 4 servings (serving size: 1/2 peach, 1/2 cup ice cream, 3 tablespoons berry sauce)

Ingredients

- 1 cup fresh berries (blackberries, raspberries, strawberries, or a combination)
- 2 tablespoons honey
- 1 tablespoon fresh lemon juice
- 1 tablespoon Grand Marnier (optional)
- 2 peaches, pitted and sliced
- 2 cups vanilla low-fat ice cream

Preparation

Combine the berries, honey, lemon juice, and Grand Marnier (if using) in a blender. Puree until smooth. Strain through a fine sieve into bowl; discard seeds and set aside. Place 4 peach slices in each of 4 dessert bowls, and add 1/2 cup ice cream to each; drizzle with berry sauce.

Nutrition: *Per serving: 189 cal, 1g fat (0.0g sat), 39g carbs, 4g fiber, 460mg sodium, 4g protein, chol 5mg*

Mini Raspberry Tarts

A tiny dessert that packs some big flavor! Low-fat dairy, like the cream cheese used in this pasty, is perfect for enjoying a tasty tart while still watching out for gout. The raspberry on top is another gout-friendly food.

Yield: Makes 32 tarts (serving size: 1 tart)

Ingredients

- 1 (16.5-ounce) package refrigerated sugar cookie dough
- 1 (8-ounce) package 1/3-less fat block-style cream cheese
- 1/4 cup sugar
- Zest of 1 orange
- 1/2 teaspoon vanilla extract
- 32 fresh raspberries

Preparation

Preheat oven to 350°. Coat a mini-muffin tin with nonstick cooking spray. Divide sugar cookie dough into 32 pieces. Coat hands in flour, and roll pieces into balls. Press each ball into tin, forming dough up and around into the shape of a tart. Bake for 11–12 minutes or until golden. Let cool 10 minutes in pan. Remove tarts, and cool completely on a wire rack. Using an electric mixer, combine cream cheese, sugar, orange zest, and vanilla. Spoon cream cheese mixture into each tart. Top each with a fresh raspberry. Chill until ready to serve.

Nutrition: *Per serving: 85 cal, 4g fat (1g sat), 11g carbs, 0g fiber, 95mg sodium, 1g protein, chol 8mg*

Vanilla Bean Pudding

Many recipes for traditional milk chocolate pudding call for thick whole milk, but by substituting it with fat-free skim milk (much better for those worried about gout) in this creamy vanilla option, you decrease the fat without sacrificing the flavor.

Vanilla beans can be expensive, but their superior flavor is worth the investment. Substitute vanilla paste or one teaspoon real vanilla extract if necessary. Stir extract in with the butter.

Yield: 6 servings (serving size: 1/2 cup)

Ingredients

- 2 1/2 cups 2% reduced-fat milk
- 1 vanilla bean, split lengthwise
- 3/4 cup sugar
- 3 tablespoons cornstarch
- 1/8 teaspoon salt
- 1/4 cup half-and-half
- 2 large egg yolks
- 4 teaspoons butter
-

Preparation

Place milk in a medium, heavy saucepan. Scrape seeds from vanilla bean; add seeds and bean to milk. Bring to a boil.

Combine sugar, cornstarch, and salt in a large bowl, stirring well. Combine half-and-half and egg yolks, stirring well. Stir egg yolk mixture into sugar mixture. Gradually add half of hot milk to sugar mixture, stirring constantly with a whisk. Return hot milk mixture to pan; bring to a boil. Cook 1 minute, stirring constantly with a whisk. Remove from heat. Add butter, stirring until melted. Remove vanilla bean; discard.

Spoon pudding into a bowl. Place bowl in a large ice-filled bowl for 15 minutes or until pudding cools, stirring occasionally. Cover surface of pudding with plastic wrap; chill.

Nutrition: *Per serving: 216 cal, 7.1g fat (4.1g sat), 34.2g carbs, 0.0g fiber, 125mg sodium, 4.6g protein, chol 86mg*

Peanut Butter Pudding Variation: Omit vanilla bean, salt, and butter; stir in 1/4 cup reduced-fat creamy peanut butter after custard is cooked. Yield: 6 servings (serving size: about 1/2 cup).

Nutrition: *Per serving: CALORIES 257 (30% from fat); FAT 8.6g (sat 3.3g, mono 3.6g, poly 1.6g); PROTEIN 6.9g; CARB 39.2g; FIBER 0.7g; CHOL*

80mg; IRON 0.5mg; SODIUM 170mg; CALC 142mg

Coconut Pudding Variation: Omit vanilla bean. Omit 3/4 cup milk, and replace it with 3/4 cup light unsweetened coconut milk. Omit butter; stir in 1/2 cup toasted sweetened flaked coconut after pudding is cooked. Yield: 6 servings (serving size: about 1/2 cup).

Nutrition: *Per serving: CALORIES 224 (30% from fat); FAT 7.5g (sat 5.3g, mono 1.5g, poly 0.4g); PROTEIN 4.1g; CARB 36.8g; FIBER 0.3g; CHOL 77mg; IRON 0.5mg; SODIUM 115mg; CALC 105mg*

Pumpkin Pancakes

You can only eat so many dense, high-calorie slices of pumpkin pie before your waistline expands. That's bad news for many reasons, including the one that being overweight can increase your risk for gout. To get that pumpkin flavor, try this 90-calorie alternative.

With these pumpkin pancakes, you can have your "cake" and eat it too!

Yield: 4 servings (serving size: about 2 pancakes, without syrup or honey)

Ingredients

- 1/2 cup canned pumpkin
- 1/2 cup low-fat vanilla yogurt
- 1/4 teaspoon baking soda
- 1 large egg yolk
- 1/4 cup cake flour
- 4 large egg whites
- 1/4 teaspoon salt
- Cooking spray
- Maple syrup or honey

Preparation

Whisk together pumpkin, yogurt, baking soda, egg yolk, and flour. Whisk egg whites with salt; fold into pumpkin mixture. Heat a large nonstick skillet coated with cooking spray over medium heat. Spoon in 1/3 cup batter for each pancake. Flip when tops are covered with bubbles and edges are slightly brown (about 3 minutes per side). Drizzle with syrup or honey.

Nutrition: *Per serving: 90 cal, 2g fat (1g sat), 12g carbs, 1g fiber, 299mg sodium, 7g protein, chol 55mg*

Cornflakes, Low-Fat Milk & Berries

Start the morning off right with this healthy bowl of cereal. Keep a bag of mixed berries in your freezer and drop them into cornflakes for a morning meal that is not only high in antioxidants and fiber, but that could also help ward off gout.

Research suggests that low-fat dairy may decrease your risk of getting gout, not to mention that dairy products are a good, meat-free source of protein.

It doesn't matter what types of berries you use for this recipe. All of them–strawberries, blueberries, raspberries, blackberries–are high in fiber, low in calories, and rich in antioxidants.

Yield: 1 serving (2 1/2 cups)

Ingredients

- 2 cups cornflakes
- 1 cup 1% low-fat milk
- 1 cup berries, fresh or frozen, thawed

Preparation

Place cornflakes in a small bowl. Top with milk and berries.

Nutrition: *Per serving: 370 cal, 3g fat (1.5g sat), 78g carbs, 6g fiber, 640mg sodium, 13g protein, chol 10mg*

9 MY GOUT HISTORY

I first acquired gout in 2007. Gout doesn't attack my toes or fingers, which is unusual, but mostly in the ankles and foot area. This occurs on both feet, but not at the same time. It seems to alternate. I've also had gout in my elbow a couple of times. My gout became so painful, that air made it hurt. Laying a sheet on it was excruciating. It amazes me to how painful it can be.

My gout attacks lasted from a couple of days to a couple of weeks. Usually once or more a month. I had a period of relief in 2011 where I was gout free for about 7 months.

I didn't realize it at the time, but my diet had changed and I had lost about 35 lbs and had become very active. This directly eliminated the gout without medication.

After a motorcycle accident, I became sedentary, gained weight and was eating fast food and comfort food. The gout came back with a fury.

I was so tired of it, that I finally decided to do something about it. I started researching as much as I could on gout. I started adopting or avoiding many of the things I learned and hence this book.

I know that obesity is the #1 culprit for me. As soon as I started losing weight, the gout became less intense and infrequent. I've been gout free for almost a year. It did require a change of lifestyle and lots of determination. Gout pain is a huge motivator. You have to change your habits and ways of thinking about nutrition, weight and exercise.

I use to eat lots of red fatty meat and drink beer. A recipe for gout. Beer is the worst. Stay away from anything with yeast.

For the first 2 months I did the following:
- Drank 2 8oz glasses of cherry juice daily
- Substituted 1 meal with a smoothie
- Stayed to low purine foods religiously.
- Avoided alcoholic drinks.
- I exercised every other day for about 30-40 minutes a day. Walking and light weights.
- Kept my caloric intake below 2000 per day.

- Maintained a daily log of what I ate.

During that period I dropped 12 lbs. I did have small gout flare ups, decreasing as I adhered to my plan. After 2 months, I was gout free. Once you have become free from gout, it's ok to have higher purine foods, but only in moderation. Moderation is the key to keeping the weight off and being gout free.

There's no big secret to this. Lose weight, eat good low purine nutrition and exercise.